Leaky Gut Syndrome

The Ultimate Cure Guide for How to Fix Your Leaky Gut Through A Leaky Gut Diet

Copyright 2015 by Wade Migan - All rights reserved.

This document is geared towards providing exact and reliable information in regards to the topic and issue covered. The publication is sold with the idea that the publisher is not required to render accounting, officially permitted, or otherwise, qualified services. If advice is necessary, legal or professional, a practiced individual in the profession should be ordered.

In no way is it legal to reproduce, duplicate, or transmit any part of this document in either electronic means or in printed format. Recording of this publication is strictly prohibited and any storage of this document is not allowed unless with written permission from the publisher. All rights reserved.

The information provided herein is stated to be truthful and consistent, in that any liability, in terms of inattention or otherwise, by any usage or abuse of any policies, processes, or directions contained within is the solitary and utter responsibility of the recipient reader. Under no circumstances will any legal responsibility or blame be held against the publisher for any reparation, damages, or monetary loss due to the information herein, either directly or indirectly.

The information herein is offered for informational purposes solely, and is universal as so. The presentation of the information is without contract or any type of guarantee assurance.

The trademarks that are used are without any consent, and the publication of the trademark is without permission or backing by the trademark owner. All trademarks and brands within this book are for clarifying purposes only and are the owned by the owners themselves, not affiliated with this document.

Table Of Contents

Introduction

Chapter 1: Understanding Leaky Gut Syndrome (LGS)

Chapter 2: Causes of Leaky Gut Syndrome

Chapter 3: Common Signs and Symptoms

Chapter 4: Testing for Leaky Gut Syndrome

Chapter 5: Managing Leaky Gut Syndrome

Chapter 6: The Leaky Gut Diet

Chapter 7: Supplements for The Leaky Gut Diet

Conclusion

Introduction

First off, I really want to thank you for downloading this book. The pages in this book were developed through years of experiences that I have gone through, as well as what has proven to work for others that I have talked to and researched. I also want to congratulate you for taking the time to understand your own leaky gut issues, and how you can overcome them through natural techniques.

The digestive system has great control over our body. From digesting food and protecting us from harmful bacteria, to transporting signals to the brain—sending physical signals, such as hunger or thirst, and emotional feelings such as stress, anxiety, joy, and even love. This multifaceted union moving through the gut is also sometimes referred to as the body's second brain, affecting our physical and psychological health.

Our digestive tract is not a "thinking brain", but it has its own senses and reflexes that work hard to keep our bodies at optimal health. It absorbs nutrients from our food intake and removes the waste from our bodies. Because of this complex system of nerves and chemicals, these exchanges of information can sometimes lead to task switching.

It isn't difficult to notice when something is wrong in our digestive tract, as changes in digestion can affect our daily lives. Whether it's abdominal cramps, diarrhea, joint pain, skin rashes, fatigue, gas, or even abdominal bloating, symptoms can be embarrassing, uncomfortable, and often weakening.

Leaky gut syndrome can be difficult to diagnose for a number of reasons: It has many different causes, it's associated with a vast array of seemingly unconnected symptoms, and evidence linking it to other health problems is unclear. However, as the evidence that this syndrome is indeed a recognizable and real condition grows, opinions are slowly changing. Eventually, leaky gut syndrome is likely to appear as one of the major medical concepts of our time.

I can guarantee that you will find this book useful if you make sure to implement what you learn in the following pages. The important thing is that you IMPLEMENT what you learn. Leaky gut syndrome is not conquered overnight, but the important thing to remember is that it is definitely possible for you to overcome it. What I am giving you is information that will enable you to understand your own situation, as well as the steps you will need to make that journey.

I recommend that you take notes while you are reading this short eBook. This will ensure that you get the most out of the information provided, and you will be able to look over the things that stuck out to you after you've finished reading. The notes will help you to pinpoint exactly what you need to implement, and by writing things down, you will be able to recall specifics and how to handle certain situations when they arise. I want you to feel that you have made a purchase well worth your money.

Lastly, remember that everything in this book has been compiled through research, my own experiences, and the experiences of others, so feel free to question what you have read in this book. I encourage you to do your own research on the things that you want to look deeper into. There are many myths created by supplement and pharmaceutical companies in order to profit off of consumers. You must be aware of what is true and false, and that is one of the reasons why I created this book.

The more you understand your own health and body, the better off you'll be. To overcome a leaky gut, it will take some work on your part, but you can do it! So remember to read with confidence and an open mind!

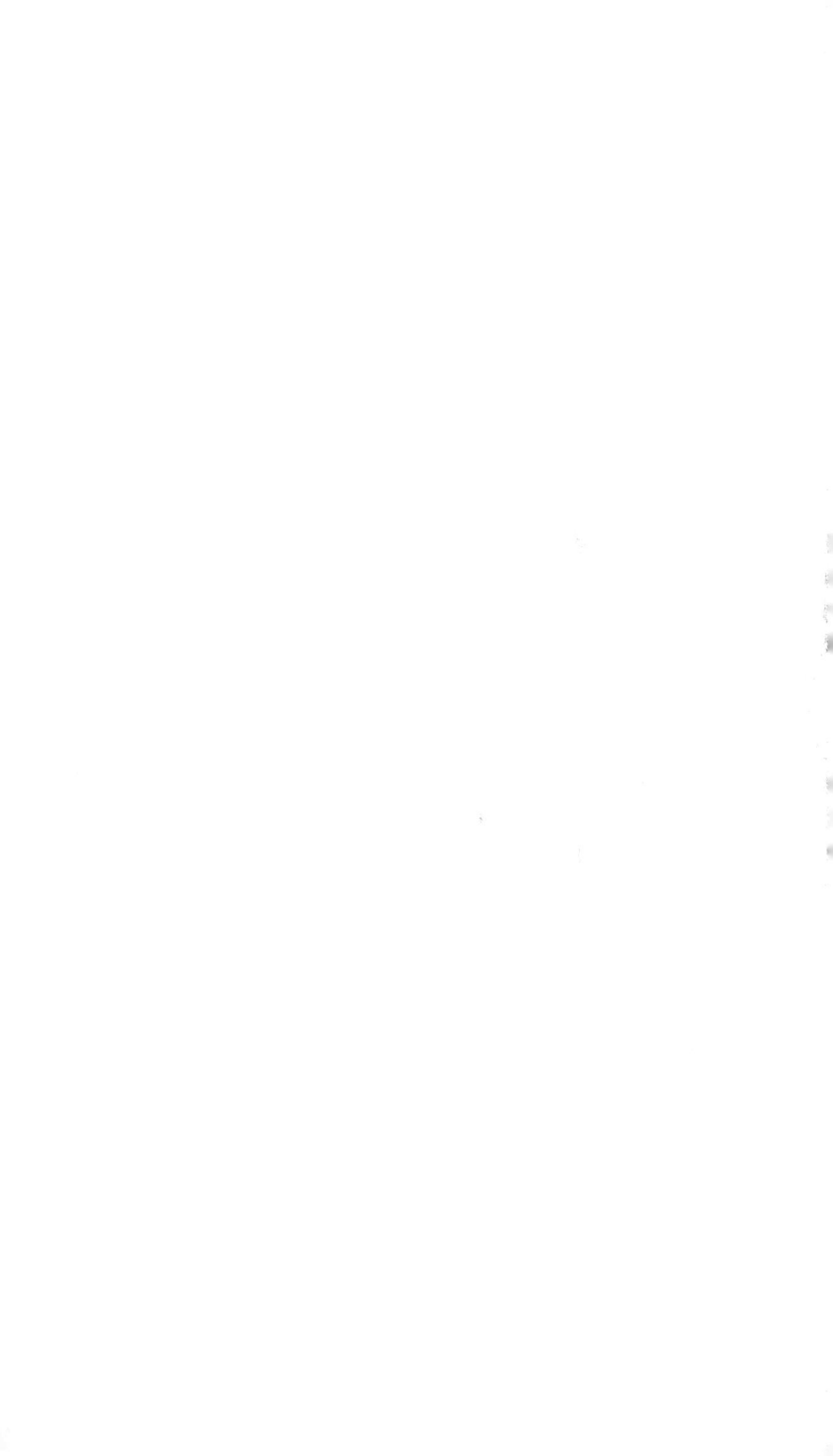

Chapter 1:

Understanding Leaky Gut Syndrome (LGS)

Leaky gut syndrome is a condition of the lower digestive tract in which the intestinal lining gets damaged. This happens when the barriers that separate pathways between the epithelial cells of the intestine break open, causing the intestinal walls to become hyperpermeable. This is why it is also referred to as "Hyperpermeable Intestines".

When this happens, the intestinal lining develops pores that are large in size, causing the undigested food molecules and some other forms of metabolic waste, such as toxins and yeast, to pass through and flow freely into the person's bloodstream.

The intestinal lining acts as the first mechanism of defense for our immune system. The epithelial cells (outer intestinal layer cells) are connected by tight junctions. At the end of these cells is something called the microvilli. These are the absorbers of the properly digested nutrients, as well as the transporters of nutrients to the epithelial cells and into the bloodstream.

In a normal digestion process, the tight junctions are closed, which force all molecules to be screened properly, so that they only pass into the bloodstream through the muscoa cells. If these tight junctions become permeable or open, they allow unscreened molecules to flow directly into the bloodstream, and it is at that point that a person can develop a leaky gut.

Initially, your body will fight any foreign element found in your blood. The liver will work extremely hard and will try to screen out all molecules that the intestinal lining was not able to screen during the first round. However, in many unfortunate cases, the liver cannot take care of all the waste in a person's bloodstream (all undigested food molecules, yeast, and toxins), because other pathogens start to multiply in the body.

Basically, the immune system will be alarmed and will fight against these foreign elements to kick them out of the body as soon as possible. However, the immune system cannot fully eliminate all these foreign elements at one time, because they are easily absorbed into all tissues throughout the body, causing them to swell or inflame.

Now that a person's body is focused on fighting these foreign elements, the little tasks, such as filtering out the blood, fighting bacteria, regulating the gut, and calming inflamed areas, are being neglected. Possible consequences of this process are:

A person's body will be fighting against itself *and* some autoimmune diseases, such as IBS, chronic fatigue, ulcerative colitis, and fibromyalgia. After that, their body will produce antibodies to fight against these foreign elements. These elements are similar to the Casein protein from milk, and other proteins from nuts, grains, or eggs.

Additionally, chemicals like Phenols and Glycerin can lead to immune responses when they enter the body. If a person's body immediately reacts to any kind of dairy product, for example, he/she will get an instant headache, sore throat, brain fog, or even sinus drainage. Similar reactions can occur if they eat foods with high Phenols content, such as tomato juice.

Finally, if a person is having sensitivities to a number of foods, it is a possibility that they are experiencing a leaky gut. Any undigested substance that is transported into the bloodstream is considered an enemy to the body by the immune system, and it will develop reactions to them that cause food intolerance. The damaged microvilli along the intestinal lining cannot produce the needed digestive enzymes to break down the food for proper digestion.

Chapter 2:

Causes of Leaky Gut Syndrome

There have been debates in the medical community about the root cause of leaky gut syndrome. However, most medical experts believe that the following are the main contributors:

Diet

Excessive intake of processed foods, preservatives, refined sugars, refined flours, and flavorings are harmful to the body. These foods have higher a content of toxins that can cause inflammation, as mentioned earlier. Additionally, the grains (such as rice, oat, and wheat) that people consume every day are also suspected to cause leaky gut syndrome. The fundamental reason of this suspicion is the high content of lectins and gliadin that are found in grains.

Chronic Stress

When you are in a chronically stressed state, your immune system will eventually get weakened. A weak immune system cannot perform its normal operations, and cannot fight pathogens effectively. This can cause gut inflammation, which can lead to increased intestinal lining permeability.

Inflammation

Any undigested food nutrients that pass through the bloodstream can cause inflammation that leads to a leaky gut. These undigested molecules can irritate everything that passes by. A leaky gut can also be caused by bacterial overgrowth, parasitic infestation, and an excessive amount of environmental toxins.

Medical Reactions

Many different types of medication, whether regulated or prohibited, can lead to a leaky gut. Pain relievers that include Aspirin or Acetaminophen can damage the intestinal lining, which inevitably leads to decreased mucosal levels (a membrane that secretes mucus on the intestinal lining). When this membrane gets compromised, the inflammation becomes severe, and more digestive issues may occur in the long run.

Yeast

Yeast is a normal habitant in the gut flora. However, when it starts to multiply rapidly, it mutates into a multi-celled fungus called Candida. Candida develops tentacles that stick on the intestinal lining, and these tentacles stay there to make holes. Eventually, the holes will serve as the exit doors of the intestinal content.

Zinc Deficiency

Zinc is a mineral that is integral in maintaining a strong intestinal lining. When the body lacks zinc, the mucosal lining will lose its strength and become more porous.

Alcohol

Drinking alcohol, particularly on an empty stomach, compromises gut health. Because of this, alcoholism makes people much more susceptible to a leaky gut.

Chapter 3:

Common Signs and Symptoms

There are various physical symptoms that point towards leaky gut syndrome. The symptoms differ from person to person, depending on the severity of the digestive tract infections. However, symptoms normally include stomach issues such as gluten intolerance, abdominal pain, and excessive bloating. It should be noted that gluten intolerance may or may not come initially.

Aside from these symptoms, any combination of the following can also happen simultaneously: Appetite loss, bladder infections, insomnia, difficulty in breathing, anxiety disorder, on-and-off fever (for no apparent cause), hemorrhoids, multiple chemical sensitivities, heartburn, malnutrition, muscle cramps, diarrhea, constipation, fatigue, anal irritations, lowered immune defenses, sluggishness, flatulence, hair loss, dull skin, brittle nails, urinary tract infection, mood swings, abdominal cramps, depression symptoms, poor memory, and anaphylactoid reactions.

Leaky gut syndrome is not a single disorder or disease. Rather, it is a cause, or side-effect, of the following diseases: Malnutrition, food allergies, giardiasis, celiac disease, asthma, liver dysfunction, irritable bowel syndrome, cystic fibrosis, crohn's disease, ulcerative colitis, colon cancer, and alcoholism. Severe medications, such as chemotherapy, can also lead to leaky gut syndrome.

It is very important to properly check the symptoms you have in order to avoid misdiagnosis and involvement in unfitting diet program. Misdiagnosis can magnify your problem.

Chapter 4:

Testing for Leaky Gut Syndrome

These days, there are several options available to test for a leaky gut, as well as related disorders or diseases. Make sure to undergo at least one of these testing options before concluding that you have a leaky gut.

Polythelyne Glycol (PEG) Test

PEG test is the most widely used method of testing for a leaky gut. The patient is given a solution containing lactulose and mannitol, and their urine is collected for testing. Lactulose (a disacharride) and mannitol (a monosacharride) are non-metabolized sugar molecules.

Mannitol is easily penetrated in cells, while lactulose contains larger molecules, hence it is partially absorbed and penetrated. Now, if the level of lactulose and mannitol in the urine sample are high, it is an indication of a leaky gut. Low levels of mannitol and high levels of lactulose indicate healthy digestion. On the other hand, low levels of both sugar molecules indicate mal-absorption of nutrients.

Digestive Stool Analysis

In this method, the patient is required to submit their stool sample to be tested. The stool will show the digestive function of the gut, by showing how well proteins, fats, and carbohydrates are absorbed in the colon. Additionally, the presence of Candida (yeast overgrowth), dysbiosis (bacterial imbalance), parasites, and other indicators of digestive dysfunction will be detected in this test.

Candida Testing

Although Candida can be detected through stool analysis, for a more thorough look it is better to perform Candida testing. This will include testing the blood for high levels of antibodies like lgA, lgG, and lgM. The presence of these three antibodies indicate Candidiasis, more commonly known as Candida.

Skin Allergy Testing/Sensitivity Testing

In addition, your doctor can also perform food allergy testing using the following methods:

Skin Prick or Scratch Test

In this test, a drop of fluid containing an allergen is put on the surface of the patient's skin (usually under the upper arm, forearm, or back arm). Then, the skin is scratched to soothe the allergen into the skin. If the patient has an allergy, his/her skin will swell and become reddish and a white wheals will develop. The swelling will fade after several hours.

Blood RAST (radioallergosorbent)

In this test, the allergen is injected underneath the surface of the patient's skin, and the reaction is closely monitored. This test is performed to measure the amount of lgE content in the patient's blood.

Patch Test

In this test, traces of allergens are taped to the patient's skin for 48 hours, then a dermatologist will measure the reaction. This is to diagnose some delayed allergic reactions that cause skin itching and rashes, such as dermatitis. Patch tests can be performed for both respiratory and food allergies.

Food Allergy/Sensitivity Testing

These are two methods used to identify food allergies:

Elimination Diet

This is a very simple method. The patient will exclude foods that are suspected to cause allergic reactions in his/her diet for several months. However, this test needs to be undertaken along with the guidance of a certified health professional.

Blood Test

This test requires the patient's blood sample to be tested for food intolerances. Upon looking at the blood-work, health professionals will be able to see what the patient is lacking and can setup a plan of how to supplement the necessary vitamins and minerals.

Live Blood Cell Analysis

Live Blood Cell Analysis requires the patient to give a pin-prick blood sample for examination. This blood sample is then placed on a microscopic slide, below the glass cover slip to prevent it from drying up. Then, the slide is examined by the practitioner using a dark field microscope (at higher magnification), and then the image is transferred to a television monitor, so that the patient can view it simultaneously.

The practitioner then evaluates the patient's state of health based on how the blood cells appear. In the monitor, the patient can see the movement of the red and white blood cells, along with the presence of toxins, bacteria, parasites, fungus, and pathogens. The practitioner can also evaluate immune system function, digestive system function, vitamin and mineral deficiencies, stresses to the system, and other indicators of diseases.

Amino Acid Analysis

Adequate consumption of amino acids are essential for optimal body functioning. The functions of amino acids are to: Produce antibodies to prevent infection, help the production of hormones such as insulin, repair muscle tissue, and carry oxygen throughout the body.

There are eight types of amino acids that the body cannot naturally produce. Malnutrition and a low protein diet can cause amino acid deficiencies. The amino acid test measures the amino acid levels in the patient's body. He/she is required to give a urine sample, and for the following 24 hours, the amino acid levels will be closely monitored by the practitioner. The test has been proven to successfully assess the risk of heart disease, digestive disorders, behavioral disorders, chronic fatigue, autism, anxiety, and fibromyalgia, among other conditions.

Chapter 5:

Managing Leaky Gut Syndrome

The medical community is not united about which particular treatment best alleviates leaky gut syndrome. Practitioners examine every possible cause of the digestive problems and address it with a patient-centered approach. They evaluate genetics, history, environment, and lifestyle factors.

There has also been scrutiny in every aspect of the treatment methods; however, the Four "R" Program has been acknowledged as a crucial tool in treating digestive disorders. This program includes: Remove, replace, reinoculate, and repair. Additionally, another "R" is being introduced into the "R" Program, and that is "regulate". This method emphasizes effective strategies to heal digestive imbalances.

Remove: Undertake a Restricted Diet

This involves eliminating sugars, grains, starches, dairy, soy, gluten, yeast, alcohol, and all other gut-irritating foods from your diet for 14 days. This is also referred to as "detox cleansing" by some people.

Initially, the elimination process will smooth and stabilize your digestive tract, which will also help to determine which foods contribute to the symptoms. It will then allow your intestinal tract to slowly return to its normal permeability, stop the free flow of foreign elements into the bloodstream, and eventually stop food intolerance symptoms.

Replace: Find Digestive Aids

Oftentimes, the conditions that lead to a leaky gut can also cause improper digestion and malabsorption, which can give you nutritional deficiencies. You need to have knowledge about the proper nutritional supplements that best support your needs. Refer to your practitioner about these.

However, in most cases, supplementing with a good multivitamin, with large amounts of Zinc and vitamin D, will help the intestinal lining to return to its normal operation. Essential fish oils have also been proven to help alleviate the condition of the intestinal mucosal lining.

Reinoculate: Rebalance Gut Flora

It is vital to keep the friendly bacteria well-balanced in your gut for optimal digestive health. Strict adherence to your restricted diet (first "R") and consumption of good bacteria, such as probiotics (Lactobacillus Acidophilus), will eventually soothe your leaky gut.

These good bacteria fight off the harmful ones (yeast and toxins) that lead to sickness and disease, heal the intestinal lining, help proper nutrients absorb, and keep the cycle on track. Additionally, fibrous foods also stabilize microbial balance. Studies have shown that maintaining a ratio of 85% good-to-bad bacteria in the gut will prevent the leaky gut syndrome from coming back.

Repair: Restore Your Intestinal Lining and Cells

There are many possible ways to rebuild, restore, and repair your intestinal lining and cells. Medical practitioners do deep research regarding ways to heal digestive disorders naturally. Their studies have shown that glutamine is helpful in keeping the proper structure and function of the intestines, and has also been shown to alleviate damage from radiation and chemotherapy.

Additionally, digestive enzymes that are found naturally in raw foods are helpful for proper digestion. They have multi-faceted abilities for soothing leaky guts. First off, they break down food into very tiny particles before they depart the stomach. This is to prevent large undigested molecules from damaging the intestinal lining and to increase nutritional absorption.

They also work as garbage collectors in your intestines by eliminating bacteria, toxins, and impaired cells of the mucosal lining. This process gives the gut a clean block of healthy cells to rebuild with. As the intestinal permeability remains, these enzymes do similar garbage collecting in the bloodstream if they are passed out of the intestinal lining. The papain and bromelain enzymes are also shown to calm inflammation in the intestinal lining and other tissues throughout the body, making the liver and the immune system reprieve.

Regulate

Finally, be aware of how you feel when you eat, where and how you eat, and, of course, what you eat. You should avoid any factors (food, toxins, etc.) that can cause negative issues in the digestive system. You should eat your meals in a relaxed setting, eat slowly, and chew your food properly. Digestion starts with an antibody in the saliva known as secretory IgA (sIgA), which is a sign of digestive immune function. Throughout the digestive tract, sIgA is the first to fight off harmful bacteria; hence, it is very important to the immune system.

Chapter 6:

The Leaky Gut Diet

The leaky gut diet is essentially a diet that is very gentle to an irritated digestive tract, and one that allows the natural healing process to occur. It includes foods that have simple nutritional content, which makes them easy to dissolve, as well as foods that have microbicidal properties.

Refer below for the types of foods that are recommended to eat, followed by other types of foods that are prohibited at all costs.

What to Eat

Eat foods that calm/sooth inflammation.

It is crucial to try to eat high amounts of both omega-3 and omega-6 fatty acids (polyunsaturated fatty acids). Omega-6 fatty acids are usually found in large quantities in modern veggies, oils, grass-fed meat, nuts, and seeds. These fatty acids are helpful because they can alleviate inflammation.

Omega-3 fatty acids that are found in pasteurized meat, pasteurized/free range eggs, and wild-caught fish can reduce inflammation. To reduce overall inflammation and heal the digestive tract, try to maintain a 1:1 ratio of omega-6 to omega-3 fatty acid intake from diet and supplementation.

In order to do this, make sure that all the meat in your diet is from grass-fed animals (beef, lamb, goat, bison, etc.); eat plenty of wild-caught fish; and/or take some natural fish oil supplements.

Additionally, vegetables are rich in vitamins, minerals, and antioxidants that calm inflammation. You need to eat various colored vegetables, and various cruciferous vegetables (broccoli, cabbage, cauliflower, kale, turnip greens, asparagus, Brussels sprouts, etc.) every day.

If you do this, you won't need to take multivitamins any longer. In this diet program, you are recommended to eat vegetables at every meal. If you miss a serving of vegetables for a meal, make it up in the following meal.

Fruits are also rich in vitamins, minerals, and antioxidants. However, in most cases, people with a leaky gut will need to minimize their intake of fruits, because of their high sugar content. It is also important that you are getting enough Vitamin D, especially if you live in a colder climate where sunlight is not abundant. You can get enough Vitamin D simply by going outside in the sun every day, from eating liver twice a week, or from taking supplements such as Cod Liver Oil and Vitamin D pills.

Eat foods that re-balance gut flora.

If your gut is irritated, chances are great that your resident good bacteria are troubled. In order to restore their population and diversity, you need to eat foods that contain probiotics.

You can do this by drinking probiotic supplements every day for a few weeks to increase the good bacteria in your body.

You can also get probiotics from unpasteurized Sauerkraut and other fermented vegetables, Kombucha tea, and coconut milk yogurt. All of these probiotic supplements can be purchased at nearby grocery stores, and some can be purchased online, but all can be made fairly easily at home.

Eat foods that encourage healing.

When your body tries to heal itself, it is crucial to provide it with foods rich in good quality protein (needed to manufacture new cells and tissues). There are several ways to achieve this; however, it is best to eat as close to paleo as possible during the healing process.

These are the recommended paleo foods that you should consume: Wild-caught fish, wild-caught sea food, grass-fed meat, organ meat (preferably from grass-fed animals), free-range eggs, and plenty of veggies.

There are two other healing foods that are also beneficial to include in your diet: Bone broth and coconut. Coconut and coconut products are rich in antimicrobial saturated fats (short and medium chain) that help decrease bad yeast production, as well as bacterial and fungus overgrowth in the small intestine.

Medium chain saturated fats are very friendly to the cells that line the digestive tract, since they can be easily absorbed without being digested by the enzymes, as well as converted into energy without any further modification. Broth that is made from the bones of beef, lamb, pork, chicken, turkey, duck, and/or fish are anti-inflammatory, anti-microbial, and help restore digestive health.

In addition to that, broth is rich in proline and glycine—amino acids that reduce inflammation, regulate digestion, and, most importantly, bring healing to every part of the body.

You may find these dietary changes overwhelming right now; however, it is important to remember that cooking your own food is beneficial, with or without leaky gut issues. Cooking your own food will save you from many diseases, as you can make sure that the food is properly cooked, and you won't have to take the risk of eating outside food that is not cooked thoroughly.

What Not to Eat

It is important to restrain yourself from eating dairy products, all grains, and all refined carbohydrates (white bread, white pasta, refined sugar, junk food, etc.) for the weeks in which you plan on fixing your leaky gut.

Furthermore, stop using monosodium glutamate (MSG), avoid additives in processed foods (many of them irritate intestinal lining), and forget using refined sugars (which cause inflammation). If possible, you should also avoid some vegetables, such as eggplants, tomatoes, potatoes, mushrooms (any fungi), and all kinds of peppers.

Starting the Leaky Gut Diet

In the first week, focus on eating the following foods: Rice, any vegetable (except tomato, potato, corn, pepper, and eggplant), quinoa millet, grass-fed meat, locally grown fruits, sunflower oil, coconut oil, olive oil, plain water, fresh organic lemon juice in water or on salads, organic green tea (if you are addicted to caffeine), and real herbal teas such as burdock, dandelion root, licorice, cleavers, red clover, meadow sweet, and nette.

If you are an athlete or you do physical labor, you need concentrated protein sources. Though these can increase food sensitivities, in most cases the gut can tolerate rice protein powder, grass-fed, hormone-free meat, and cold-water ocean fish.

If you experience a "detox" reaction during the first 24-48 hours in the first week, don't stress out—this is normal. You may feel a slight fever, but it will pass quickly if you drink enough water, rest, and strictly follow your leaky gut diet. Castor oil packs, saunas, and Epsom salt baths can also ease the detox process.

The leaky gut diet is most effective if you continue for two to four weeks consistently. After that, your leaky gut issues should be resolved; however, you can still make long-term adjustments to your diet using some of the guidelines presented in this book.

Chapter 7:

Supplements for The Leaky Gut Diet

There are various supplements that can help restore your digestive health, but the most beneficial are the following:

L-Glutamine

Glutamine is an important amino acid that is anti-inflammatory and essential for the growth and repair of your digestive tract. L-Glutamine acts as a repellant to irritants and protects and coats the cell walls.

Digestive Enzymes

Digestive enzymes ensure that the foods you eat are properly digested, reducing the chance that partially digested food molecules will damage your intestinal lining. It is advised to take 1 to 2 capsules of digestive enzymes each day in your recovery process.

Aloe Vera

Aloe Vera helps the healing of ulceritis and other injuries in the digestive tract. It also helps the healing of burns within the body.

Licorice Root and Slippery Elm

Licorice root, slippery elm, and other demulcent herbs calm the mucus membranes that line the digestive tract; they act as a bandage. Other herbs, like peppermint and ginger, can also sooth inflammation because of their anti-inflammatory properties.

Probiotics

As mentioned earlier, probiotics are a crucial factor in healing your leaky gut. You can get probiotics in food and/or supplement form, depending on your personal preference.

Most people only follow part of the protocol in healing their leaky gut, by eliminating the damaging irritants—the part they always seem to leave out is rebalancing their gut with *friendly* bacteria that will fight off *harmful* bacteria. So, eat a lot of probiotic-rich foods and, if you choose the supplement route, go with a high quality brand.

Conclusion

I worked hard on creating the best guide for "overcoming leaky gut syndrome" that I could. These are all the strategies and information that has worked for me, as well as others that I have talked to and researched. I guarantee that if you stay consistent, they will work for you as well. Be optimistic about your current situation and make small progress each day!

The next step is to see your doctor or health care provider before engaging yourself in the leaky gut diet. Though the leaky gut diet has been proven effective in treating leaky gut syndrome, it is essential to consult with your doctor for proper diagnosis and treatment, because symptoms can vary from person to person. Make sure to undergo the different testing procedures in order to identify the root cause of your digestive issues.

If you feel like you learned something from this book, please take the time to share your thoughts with me by sending me a message or by leaving a review on Amazon. It would be greatly appreciated!

Thank you and good luck on your journey!

Printed in Great Britain
by Amazon.co.uk, Ltd.,
Marston Gate.